OTHER BOOKS BY LUCINDA GIBBS ROBINSON

NATURAL HERBAL THERAPY
(A Scriptural based step by step plan to cure yourself of AIDS, cancer, and many other health challenges)

HOW TO STOP ALCOHOL CRAVINGS

SHOT DETOX

DETOX YOUR BODY FROM VACCINATIONS, IMMUNIZATIONS, AND FLU SHOTS EVEN YEARS AFTER TAKING THEM

AND

HELP STRENGTHEN AND HEAL YOUR CHILDREN AFTER SHOTS

BY

LUCINDA GIBBS ROBINSON

2017

Revised 2021

MY NAME IS LUCINDA GIBBS ROBINSON. I AM AN HERBALIST SINCE 1973, EDUCATING PEOPLE ABOUT NATURAL, NON-INVASIVE WAYS TO OVERCOME MANY HEALTH PROBLEMS NATURALLY. MY SIMPLIFIED, STEP BY STEP BOOK ON ACHIEVING AND RECLAIMING HEALTH NATURALLY IS NAMED NATURAL HERBAL THERAPY.

I TEACH ABOUT THE IMMUNE SYSTEM AND HOW TO BUILD IT UP NATURALLY. I TEACH ABOUT HOW PEOPLE GET SICK AND HOW TO GET WELL NATURALLY. I TEACH ABOUT ORGANIC AND RAW FOODS FOR EXCELLENT HEALTH. I TEACH ABOUT HERBS, ESSENTIAL OILS, ORGANIC JUICES, AND THEIR MEDICINAL PROPERTIES. I TEACH ABOUT NORMALIZING THE BODY'S CHEMICAL PROCESSES WITH ENZYMES, PROBIOTICS, MINERALS, AND VITAMINS. I TEACH HOW TO DETOX FROM UNNATURAL SUBSTANCES THAT ARE IN YOUR BODY.

I HAVE DEVELOPED SUCCESSFUL, INDIVIDUALIZED REGIMENS FOR HUNDREDS OF PEOPLE TO OVERCOME AND TOTALLY RECOVER FROM AIDS, CANCER, DIABETES, ASTHMA, KIDNEY DISEASE, MULTIPLE SCLEROSIS, LYME DISEASE, FIBRAMYRALGIA, AND MANY OTHER DISEASES AND CONDITIONS USING ONLY ORGANIC FOODS, HERBS, JUICES, VITAMINS AND MINERALS, ENZYMES, PROBIOTICS, ESSENTIAL OILS, SEA VEGETABLES, EARTH CLAYS, EARTH MATERIALS, CHARCOALS, DIFFERENT NATURAL

SALTS- ALL ORGANIC, ALL NATURAL AGENTS OF HEALING.

I HELP PREGNANT MOTHERS BY DESIGNING FULL PRENATAL REGIMENS TO HELP THEM FORM INTELLIGENT, WELL FORMED, BEAUTIFUL, CALM, HAPPY, AND HEALTHY BABIES.

IN RECENT YEARS...AND REACHING POSSIBLY FAR INTO THE FUTURE... I SEE A NEW KIND OF DECEPTION LEADING INTO A NEW KIND OF HEALTH HOLOCAUST...IN THE DAMAGING OF OUR BABIES, CHILDREN, AND ADULTS BY VACCINATIONS, IMMUNIZATIONS, AND FLU SHOTS. IT IS SO EVIL AND PERNICIOUS. AT THIS POINT, MILLIONS OF US HAVE ALREADY BEEN DAMAGED, AND SOME EVEN HAVE DIED.

BUT YOU ALREADY KNOW THAT OR YOU WOULD NOT BE READING THIS BOOK.....

I WILL MAKE IT SHORT. THERE IS A VAST AMOUNT OF INFORMATION ON THE INTERNET ON THIS TOPIC LISTED AT THE END OF THIS BOOK. THERE IS A LIST OF INTERNET SITES THAT HAVE ALL THE FACTS.

MY PURPOSE IN THIS BOOK IS TO SHOW YOU HOW TO DETOX FROM THESE INJECTIONS AND GET WELL AGAIN- EVEN AFTER MANY YEARS OF SUFFERING FROM THE EFFECTS OF THE CHEMICALS AND FILTH IN THESE INJECTIONS.

THE CHEMICALS THAT ACCOMPANY THE SUPPOSED "HEALTH" BUILDING INGREDIENTS OF VACCINES ARE DEADLY AND MAIMING AND FILTHY. AND THE SUPPOSED "HEALTH" BUILDING AGENTS ARE ALIVE AND INFECTIVE, MANY TIMES GIVING YOU THE ACTUAL DISEASE YOU ARE SUPPOSEDLY TRYING TO PREVENT! AND ALSO MAKING YOU A ONE PERSON MANURE TYPE SPREADER OF INFECTION OF THAT VERY DISEASE TO THOSE AROUND YOU!

IF YOU BELIEVE IN THE BIBLE AND ITS INSTRUCTIONS FOR HEALTH AND HOLINESS, THERE IS NO WAY YOU CAN TAKE ANY OF THESE INJECTIONS OR ALLOW YOUR CHILDREN TO TAKE THEM. THEY CONTAIN MANY SCRIPTURALLY UNCLEAN THINGS AS OUTLINED IN LEVITICUS 11 AND DEUTERONOMY 14.

I WANT YO GIVE YOU A STEP BY STEP PLAN TO REMOVE AS MANY OF THESE HARMFUL SUBSTANCES AS POSSIBLE AS QUICKLY AS POSSIBLE.

THE SOONER YOU DETOX AFTER THE INJECTION, THE BETTER. BUT DOING IT EVEN AFTER MANY YEARS CAN STILL HELP RELIEVE SOME OR ALL OF THE SYMPTOMS YOU HAVE EXPERIENCED.

WHAT WE KNOW FOR SURE-

Other countries outside of the USA have proven through their research and courts that these injections and their ingredients cause newly formed diseases and conditions.

At approximately the same time vaccinations were first introduced, greatly improved sanitary conditions had nearly eradicated all the diseases that we are now being told for which we must be vaccinated. Inside clean water flushing toilets, municipal water filtering systems, underground, enclosed septic and sewer systems, indoor running water, washing machines, high temperature clothes dryers, high temperature dishwashers, hot water heaters, indoor showers, refrigerators and freezers to keep foods from spoiling, the sterilization of reusable medical/surgical equipment, the iron and washable cover ironing board, disposable toilet tissue, disposable nasal/facial tissue, disposable dinner napkins, disposable sanitary napkins, disposable paper towels, disposable sponges, the wearing of gloves in medical procedures, window screening, the wearing of washable cotton gloves in social occasions, the raising of hems to above the street level of women's dresses so that animal manures would not be dragged into homes, outside spigots on homes to wash off dirt and leave it outside the home, mosquito netting, the drinking of quinine water-all things that washed or disinfected or kept pathogens AWAY from other humans and more all contributed to the drastic reduction in diseases being spread.

VACCINATIONS, IMMUNIZATIONS, AND FLU SHOTS...

HISTORY

Enter Dr. Jonas Salk and the race to develop a commercially viable polio vaccine. Salk and his peers concocted a vaccine from a mad scientist brew of ingredients including **the minced up spinal cord from a 9-year-old deceased patient, water, blood, flies, feces, and human cell matter**. This mixture was injected into the brains of monkeys, most of which died instantly or became paralyzed.

Learn more:

www.naturalnews.com/033834_vaccines_ingredients.html

Undaunted, Salk plugged away eventually creating the commercial version of the polio vaccine, developed in part from "the feces of three healthy children in Cleveland."

Learn more:

www.naturalnews.com/033834_vaccines_ingredients.html

While today's formulations AS FAR AS WE KNOW don't contain feces, they are still derived from live hosts including cows, monkeys, pigs, chicken embryos, and human diploid cells harvested from aborted babies' body parts, and other filth.

Learn more:

www.naturalnews.com/033834_vaccines_ingredients.html

"Vaccines are not filtered clean, but suspension from the manufacturers' incubation tanks in which the viruses are produced from substrates of mashed bird embryo, minced monkey kidneys, or the infamous cloned human diploid cells (from aborted babies' body parts) only scanned for a few known contaminates - while the unknowns remain just that -- unknown."

Learn more:
www.naturalnews.com/033834_vaccines_ingredients.html

In the beginning of educating the public about the "necessity" of vaccinations, we were told that a vaccine was prepared by killing live pathogens and suspending them in a solution to be injected into the body so that ANTIBODIES could be formed against these "dead" pathogens. Unfortunately, not all the pathogens were killed. Many live pathogens survived actually giving the receiver of the vaccine the very disease it was supposed to prevent!

ANTIBODIES CAN ONLY BE FORMED AGAINST VIRUSES. SO ANY VACCINATION AGAINST A BACTERIA, MOLD, FUNGI, OR PARASITE IS ABSOLUTELY WORTHLESS AND EXTREMELY DECEIVING!

VACCINE INGREDIENTS

Vaccines contain ingredients such as:

monosodium glutamate (MSG),

antifreeze (deadly, causes kidney failure, intoxication),

phenol (used as VERY STRONG disinfectant),

formaldehyde (cancer causing and used to embalm the dead),

aluminum (associated with Alzheimer's disease and seizures),

glycerin (toxic to the kidney, liver, can cause lung damage, gastrointestinal damage and death),

lead (deadly ONCE IT CROSSES THE BLOOD BRAIN BARRIER),

cadmium (TOXIC TO HUMANS IN EVEN MINUTE AMOUNTS,

sulfates (SAME AS ACID RAIN),

yeast proteins,

antibiotics (can cause severe allergic reactions),

acetone (used in nail polish remover, flammable, volatile),

neomycin (causes kidney damage, tinnitus), and

streptomycin (causes fetal auditory toxicity and neuromuscular paralysis, kidney and ear toxicity, tinnitus, vertigo, ataxia, vomiting, numbness, fever, rash) ,

sucrose (gout, obesity, diabetes),

fructose (gout, liver function),

dextrose (ADDICTIVE AS COCAINE),

potassium phosphate (fertilizer, foaming agent),

FD&C Yellow #6,

aluminum lake dye (DAMAGES BRAIN),

fetal bovine serum (from dead cow fetus),

sodium bicarbonate (leavening agent),

aluminum hydroxide (CAUSES NEUROLOGICAL DISORDERS),

benzethonium chloride (antimicrobial),

lactose (cow milk sugar),

aluminum potassium sulfate (COMMERCIAL FERTILIZER),

peptone (digested animal tissue),

bovine extract (any number of cow organs extract),

thimerosal (CAUSES MERCURY POISONING, nerve damage, toxic, AUTISM, AUTISTIC SPECTRUM DISORDERS), ammonium sulfate (fertilizer, insecticide),

glutaraldehyde (disinfectant, fixative),

calf serum (dead calf extract),

aluminum phosphate (BRAIN DISORDERS, fertilizer),

aluminum hydroxphosphate sulfate (fertilizer),

ethanol (neurotoxic and psychoactive drug),

vero cell culture (monkey kidney cells),

mouse serum protein (mouse brain material),

human serum albumin (human blood tissue),

gelatin (from pig, cow, or horse bones),

HUMAN DIPLOID CELLS (HARVESTED FROM ABORTED BABIES' BODY PARTS!!), etc.

No one knows exactly how deadly injecting into the flesh it is to allow animal DNA, another human's DNA, opposite sex human DNA, animal urine, plus many, many heavy metals and pollutant chemicals singly, and certainly not in multiples, to enter the tissues without it being FULLY BROKEN DOWN firstly through the digestive system, let alone directly injected!

Some of the animal tissue and cells injected are from Scripturally unclean animals, something strictly forbidden by the Creator of us all! Leviticus 11 and Deuteronomy 14 EXPLAINS

THE USE OF UNCLEAN ANIMALS WITHIN THE HUMAN BODY WITH THE STRONGEST WORD OF DISGUST IN THE HEBREW LANGUAGE- ABOMINATION! And the horrific act of injecting it or another human's DNA into the flesh is way beyond the conscience of most thinking individuals.

WHAT WE DO KNOW IS THAT------

*THE MORE VACCINATIONS SOMEONE GETS, THE MORE LIKELY THE MORE HEALTH PROBLEMS HE HAS.

*THE MORE VACCINATIONS SOMEONE GETS, THE MORE LIKELY THEY WILL HAVE LONG TERM HEALTH PROBLEMS.

*THE MORE VACCINATIONS THEY RECEIVE, THE MORE LIKELY THE MORE HEALTH PROBLEMS MULTIPLY AFTER EACH NEXT VACCINATION.

*AND THE MORE VACCINATIONS SOMEONE GETS, THE MORE LIKELY THEY WILL DIE SOON AFTER THE NEXT ONE!

*AND THE MORE VACCINATIONS ANYONE GETS AT ONE TIME, THE MORE LIKELY THEY WILL DIE WITHIN 3 DAYS OF THE VACCINATIONS!

Learn more:

www.naturalnews.com/047167_vaccines_heavy_metals_detoxification.html

This is a list of vaccination ingredients of vaccinations most commonly used in the USA. This list is from Wikipedia updated on 10/4/2016. This list is identical with the list released by the CDC- Center for Disease Control.

Vaccine	Culture media	Excipients
Adenovirus vaccine	Dulbecco's Modified Eagle Medium, human diploid fibroblast cell culture (WI-38)	Acetone, alcohol, anhydrous lactose, castor oil, cellulose acetate phthalate, dextrose, D-fructose, D-mannose, FD&C Yellow #6 aluminum lake dye, fetal bovine serum, human serum albumin, magnesium stearate, micro crystalline cellulose, plasdone C, Polacrilin potassium, potassium phosphate, sodium bicarbonate, sucrose
Anthrax vaccine (Biothrax)	Puziss-Wright medium 1095, synthetic or semisynthetic	Aluminum hydroxide, amino acids, benzethonium chloride, formaldehyde, inorganic salts and sugars, vitamins
BCG (Bacillus Calmette-Guérin) (TICE BCG)	Synthetic or semisynthetic	Asparagine, citric acid, lactose, glycerin, iron ammonium citrate, magnesium sulfate, potassium phosphate
DTaP (DAPTACEL)	Cohen-Wheeler or Stainer-Scholte media, synthetic or semisynthetic	Aluminum phosphate, formaldehyde, Glutaraldehyde, 2-phenoxyethanol
DTaP (Infanrix)	Cohen-Wheeler or Stainer-Scholte media, Lathan medium derived from bovine casein, Linggoud-Fenton medium derived from bovine extract, synthetic or semisynthetic	Aluminum hydroxide, bovine extract, formaldehyde, glutaraldhyde, polysorbate 80
DTaP (Tripedia)	Cohen-Wheeler or Stainer-Scholte media, synthetic or semisynthetic	Aluminum potassium sulfate, ammonium sulfate, bovine extract, formaldehyde, gelatin, peptone, polysorbate 80, sodium phosphate, thimerosal[2]
DTaP/Hib (TriHIBit)	Synthetic or semisynthetic	Aluminum potassium sulfate, ammonium sulfate, bovine extract, formaldehyde or formalin, gelatin, polysorbate 80, sucrose, thimerosal[2]
DTaP-IPV (KINRIX)	Vero (monkey kidney) cell culture, synthetic or semisynthetic	Aluminum hydroxide, calf serum, formaldehyde, glutaraldehyde, lactalbumin hydrolysate, neomycin sulfate, polymyxin B, polysorbate 80

Vaccine	Growth Medium	Other Ingredients
DTaP-HepB-IPV (Pediarix)	Bovine protein, Lathan medium derived from bovine casein, Linggoud-Fenton medium derived from bovine extract, Vero (monkey kidney) cell culture, synthetic or semisynthetic	Aluminum hydroxide, aluminum phosphate, calf serum, lactalbumin hydrolysate, formaldehyde, glutaraldhyde, neomycin sulfate, polymyxin B, polysorbate 80, yeast protein
DtaP-IPV/Hib (Pentacel)	Synthetic or semisynthetic	Aluminum phosphate, bovine serum albumin, formaldehyde, glutaraldehyde, MRC-5 cellular protein, neomycin, polymyxin B sulfate, polysorbate 80, 2-phenoxyethanol
DT (diphtheria vaccine plus tetanus vaccine) (Sanofi)	Synthetic or semisynthetic	Aluminum potassium sulfate, bovine extract, formaldehyde, thimerosal
DT (Massachusetts)	Synthetic or semisynthetic	Aluminum hydroxide, formaldehyde or formalin
Hib vaccine (ActHIB)	Synthetic or semisynthetic	Ammonium sulfate, formaldehyde, sucrose
Hib (PedvaxHib)	Synthetic or semisynthetic	Aluminum hydroxyphosphate sulfate
Hib (Hiberix)	Semisynthetic	Formaldehyde, lactose
Hib/Hep B (Comvax)	Synthetic or semisynthetic, yeast or yeast extract	Amorphous aluminum hydroxyphosphate sulfate, amino acids, dextrose, formaldehyde, hemin chloride, mineral salts, nicotinamide adenine dinucleotide, potassium aluminum sulfate, sodium borate, soy peptone, yeast protein
Hepatitis A vaccine (Havrix)	Human diploid tissue culture (MRC-5)	Aluminum hydroxide, amino acid supplement, formalin, MRC-5 cellular protein, neomycin sulfate, phosphate buffers, polysorbate 20
Hepatitis A vaccine (VAQTA)	Human diploid tissue culture (MRC-5)	Amorphous aluminum hydroxyphosphate sulfate, bovine albumin or serum, formaldehyde, MRC-5 cellular protein, sodium borate
Hepatitis B vaccine (Engerix-B)	Yeast or yeast extract	Aluminum hydroxide, phosphate buffers, yeast protein
Hepatitis B vaccine (Recombivax HB)	Yeast or yeast extract	Amorphous aluminum hydroxyphosphate sulfate, amino acids, dextrose, formaldehyde, mineral salts, potassium aluminum sulfate, soy peptone, yeast protein
HepA/HepB	Human diploid tissue culture	Aluminum hydroxide, aluminum phosphate,

vaccine (Twinrix)	(MRC-5), yeast or yeast extract	amino acids, formalin, MRC-5 cells, neomycin sulfate, phosphate buffers, polysorbate 20, yeast protein
Human papillomavirus (HPV) (Cervarix)	*Trichoplusia ni* cells	Aluminum hydroxide, amino acids, lipids, mineral salts, sodium dihydrogen phosphate dehydrate, type 16 viral protein L1, type 18 viral protein L1, vitamins
Human papillomavirus (HPV) (Gardasil)	Yeast or yeast extract	Amino acids, amorphous aluminum hydroxyphosphate sulfate, carbohydrates, L-histidine, mineral salts, polysorbate 80, sodium borate, vitamins, yeast protein
Influenza vaccine (Afluria)	Chicken embryo	Beta-propiolactone, calcium chloride, dibasic sodium phosphate, egg protein, monobasic potassium phosphate, monobasic sodium phosphate, neomycin sulfate, polymyxin B, potassium chloride, sodium taurodeoxychoalate, thimerosal (multi-dose vials only)
Influenza vaccine (Agriflu)	Chicken embryo	Egg proteins, formaldehyde, polysorbate 80, cetyltrimethylammonium bromide, neomycin sulfate, kanamycin
Influenza vaccine (Fluarix)	Chicken embryo	Formaldehyde, octoxynol-10 (Triton X-100), α-tocopheryl hydrogen succinate, polysorbate 80 (Tween 80), hydrocortisone, gentamicin sulfate, ovalbumin, sodium deoxycholate, sucrose, phosphate buffer
Influenza vaccine (Flublok)	insect cell line (expresSF+®)	Monobasic sodium phosphate, dibasic sodium phosphate, polysorbate 20, baculovirus and host cell proteins, baculovirus and cellular DNA, Triton X-100, lipids, vitamins, amino acids, mineral salts
Influenza vaccine (Flucelvax)	Madin Darby Canine Kidney (MDCK) cell protein	Madin Darby Canine Kidney (MDCK) cell protein, MDCK cell DNA, polysorbate 80, cetyltrimethlyammonium bromide, β-propiolactone, phosphate buffer
Influenza vaccine (Flulaval)	Chicken embryo	Formaldehyde, á-tocopheryl hydrogen succinate, polysorbate 80, sodium deoxycholate, thimerosal, ovalbumin
Influenza vaccine (Fluvirin)	Chicken embryo	Beta-propiolactone, egg protein, neomycin, nonylphenol ethoxylate, polymyxin, thimerosal (multi-dose containers), thimerosal[2] (single-dose syringes)
Influenza vaccine	Chicken embryo	Egg protein, formaldehyde, gelatin (standard

(Fluzone)		formulation only), octylphenol ethoxylate (Triton X-100), sodium phosphate, thimerosal (multi-dose containers only)
Influenza vaccine (FluMist)	Chicken kidney cells, chicken embryo	Arginine, dibasic potassium phosphate, egg protein, ethylenediaminetetraacetic acid, gentamicin sulfate, hydrolyzed porcine gelatin, monobasic potassium phosphate, monosodium glutamate, sucrose
Japanese encephalitis vaccine (JE-Vax)	Mouse brain culture	Formaldehyde or formalin, gelatin, mouse serum protein, polysorbate 80, thimerosal
Japanese encephalitis vaccine (Ixiaro)	Vero (monkey kidney) cell culture	Aluminum hydroxide, bovine serum albumin, formaldehyde, protamine sulfate, sodium metabisulphite
Meningococcal vaccine (Menactra)	Modified Mueller-Miller medium, Mueller Hinton agar, Watson Scherp medium	Formaldehyde (Each 0.5 mL dose may contain residual amounts of formaldehyde of less than 2.66 µg (0.000532%), by calculation), phosphate buffers[3]
Meningococcal vaccine (Menomune)	Watson Scherp media, Mueller Hinton agar	Lactose, thimerosal (multi-dose vial only)
Meningococcal vaccine (Menveo)	Franz complete medium	Amino acids, formaldehyde, yeast extract
MMR vaccine (MMR-II)	Human diploid tissue culture (WI-38), Medium 199	Amino acids, fetal bovine serum, glutamate, hydrolyzed gelatin, neomycin, recombinant human serum albumin, sodium phosphate, sorbitol, sucrose, vitamins
MMRV vaccine (ProQuad)	Human diploid tissue cultures (MRC-5, WI-38), Medium 199	Bovine calf serum, dibasic potassium phosphate, dibasic sodium phosphate, human albumin, human serum albumin, hydrolyzed gelatin, monobasic potassium phosphate, monosodium L-glutamate, MRC-5 cellular protein, neomycin, sodium bicarbonate, sorbitol, sucrose, potassium chloride
Pneumococcal vaccine (Pneumovax)	Bovine protein	Phenol
Pneumococcal vaccine (Prevnar)	Soy peptone broth	Aluminum phosphate, ammonium sulfate, casamino acid, polysorbate 80, succinate buffer, yeast
Polio vaccine (IPV - IPOL)	Vero (monkey kidney) cell culture, Medium 199	Calf serum protein, formaldehyde, neomycin, 2-phenoxyethanol, polymyxin B,

		streptomycin
Polio vaccine (IPV - Poliovax)	Human diploid tissue culture (MRC-5)	sodium chloride
Rabies vaccine (Imovax)	Human diploid tissue culture (MRC-5)	Albumin, MRC-5 cells, neomycin sulfate, phenol
Rabies vaccine (RabAvert)	Rhesus fetal lung tissue culture, chicken embryo	Amphotericin B, beta-propiolactone, chicken protein, chlortetracycline, human serum albumin, neomycin, ovalbumin, polygeline (processed bovine 14 gelatin), potassium glutamate
Rotavirus vaccine (RotaTeq)	Vero (monkey kidney) cell culture	fetal bovine serum, sodium citrate, sodium phosphate monobasic monohydrate, sodium hydroxide, sucrose, polysorbate 80
Rotavirus vaccine (ROTARIX)	Dulbecco's Modified Eagle Medium (DMEM)	Amino acids, calcium carbonate, dextran, sorbitol, sucrose, vitamins, xanthan
Td vaccine (Decavac)	Mueller & Miller medium, synthetic or semisynthetic	Aluminum potassium sulfate, bovine muscle tissue, formaldehyde, peptone, thimerosal[2]
Td vaccine (Mass)	Modified Mueller's media, synthetic or semisynthetic	Aluminum phosphate, ammonium phosphate, bovine extracts, formaldehyde, thimerosal (some multi-dose vials)
Tdap vaccine (Adacel)	Mueller's growth medium, Mueller-Miller casamino acidmedium(without beef heart infusion), synthetic or semisynthetic	Aluminum phosphate, ammonium sulfate, formaldehyde, glutaraldehyde, 2-phenoxyethanol
Tdap vaccine (Boostrix)	Fenton media with bovine casein, Lathan medium derived from bovine casein, Linggoud-Fenton medium derived from bovine extract, Stainer-Scholte liquid medium, synthetic or semisynthetic	Aluminum hydroxide, bovine extract, formaldehyde, glutaraldehyde, polysorbate 80
Typhoid vaccine (inactivated – TYPHIM Vi)	Synthetic or semisynthetic	Disodium phosphate, monosodium phosphate, phenol, polydimethylsiloxane, hexadecyltrimethylammonium bromide
Typhoid vaccine (oral – Ty21a/Vivotif)		Amino acids, ascorbic acid, casein, dextrose, galactose, lactose, sucrose, yeast extract
Vaccinia (ACAM2000)	Vero (monkey kidney) cell culture	Glycerin, human serum albumin, mannitol, neomycin, phenol, polymyxin B

Varicella vaccine (Varivax)	Human diploid tissue cultures (MRC-5 and WI-38)	Dibasic sodium phosphate, ethylenediamine tetra acetic acid[sodium (EDTA), fetal bovine serum, gelatin, glutamate, monobasic potassium phosphate, monobasic sodium phosphate, monosodium L-glutamate, MRC-5 DNA and cellular protein, neomycin, phosphate, potassium chloride, sucrose
Yellow fever vaccine (YF-Vax)	Chicken embryo	Egg protein, gelatin, sorbitol
Zoster vaccine (Zostavax)	Human diploid tissue cultures (MRC-5 and WI-38)	Bovine calf serum, dibasic sodium phosphate, hydrolyzed porcine gelatin, monosodium L-glutamate, MRC-5 DNA and cellular protein, monobasic potassium phosphate, neomycin, potassium chloride, sucrose

NATURAL AGENTS THAT DETOX VACCINATIONS, IMMUNIZATIONS, AND FLU SHOTS

These should be used as the mainstay of your diet during the time of your shot detoxification! EVERYTHING I LIST IN THIS BOOK IN ANY FORM IS ALWAYS ORGANIC! The things mentioned in these lists are easily available in North America.

- ACAI FRUIT
- ARTICHOKES
- ASPARAGUS
- AVOCADO
- BEETS
- BENTONITE CLAY
- BERGAMOT FRUIT
- BLACK GRAPES
- BROCCOLI, BROCCOLINI, RAPINI, RAPE GREENS
- BRUSSEL SPROUTS
- BURDOCK ROOT TEA
- CABBAGE-ALL KINDS -GREEN, SAVOY, CHINESE, PURPLE
- CANNABIS OIL- HIGH CBD
- CARROT JUICE-ALL COLORS
- CAULIFLOWER
- CILANTRO
- CINNAMON CEYLONICUM OR ZEYLONICUM
- CITRUS AND CITRUS PEELS- LEMON, LIME, GRAPEFRUIT, ORANGE, TANGERINE, BERGAMOT
- CHARCOAL

- CHLORELLA
- COCONUT OIL
- CONCORD GRAPES
- DANDELION GREENS AND TEA
- DIATOMACEOUS EARTH
- FLAXSEED AND FLAXSEED FIBER
- GARLIC
- GINGER
- GLUTATHIONE
- GOGI FRUIT
- GOLDENSEAL TEA
- GREENS JUICE
- GREEN TEA
- KALE
- KELPS OF ALL KINDS
- LEEKS
- LEMONGRASS
- LICORICE
- MANGOSTEEN FRUIT
- MUSCADINE GRAPES
- NONI FRUIT
- NUTS OF ANY KIND-WALNUTS, ALMONDS, BRAZIL, HAZELNUTS, PECANS
- OLIVES AND OLIVE OIL
- ONIONS OF ALL KINDS
- OREGANO
- PARSLEY
- POMEGRANATE
- PSYLLIUM SEED AND FIBER
- PUMPKIN SEED AND FIBER
- PURPLE GRAPES

- ROSEMARY
- SCUPPERNOGG GRAPES
- SEAWEEDS/SEAGREENS OF ALL KINDS
- SEEDS OF ANY KIND- HEMP, SUNFLOWER, CHIA, SESAME, BLACK
- SOURSOP FRUIT
- SPIRULINA
- TUMERIC
- WATER
- WATERCRESS
- WHEATGRASS AND WHEATGRASS JUICE

Moringa and frankincense can unscramble damaged DNA- absolute musts in dealing with autism and autistic spectrum disorders.

Garlic can repair damaged nerves.

B-100 complex and multiform magnesium can provide nerves with missing nutrients to function normally.

Lemongrass oil, pine needle oil, spruce oils, cypress oils, and lemon or other citrus oils can dismantle longstanding viruses.

Cilantro and burdock root eliminate mercury, nickel, tin, and aluminum from your body.

HERBS-

BITTERSWEET
BLOODROOT
BLUE COHOSH
BLUE FLAG
BORAGE
BURDOCK ROOT
CHICKWEED
CILANTRO
CINNAMON ZEYLONICUM
CLEAVERS
DANDELION ROOT
ECHINACEA
ELDER
ELECAMPANE
FIREWEED
FRINGE TREE
GARLIC
GENTIAN ROOT
GINGER
GOLDEN SEAL ROOT AND LEAF
GOLDENTHREAD
HOLY THISTLE
HORSETAIL
HYSSOP
LEMON
LEMONGRASS
MYRRH
NETTLE
OREGANO

PARSLEY
PINE NEEDLE
PLANTAIN
PRICKLY ASH
RED CLOVER
ROSEMARY
SAINT JOHN'S WORT
SANICLE
SARSAPARILLA
SASSAFRAS
SLIPPERY ELM
SMART WEED
SORREL
SPIKENARD
TUMERIC
TURKEY CORN
WATER PEPPER
WHITE CLOVER
WILD OREGON GRAPE
YELLOW DOCK

ESSENTIAL OILS

NEARLY ANY ESSENTIAL OIL FACILITATES THE EXIT OF HARMFUL SUBSTANCES FROM THE BODY. THE HIGHER THE VIBRATIONAL QUALITIES OF THE INDIVIDUAL ESSENTIAL OIL, THE MORE EFFECTIVE IT IS AT DETOXIFYING MORE VARIETIES OF PATHOGENS. I LIKE TO EXPLAIN IT IN LECTURES AS – THE HIGHER THE FREQUENCY, THE BIGGER THE UMBRELLA OF PROTECTION AGAINST A GREATER NUMBER OF PATHOGENS!

These oils should be rubbed on the backs of infants so that they can not reach the oil with their hands and get them in their eyes. Adults may rub them on their skin, feet, or take several drops of any in an empty veggie capsule.

- Rose (Rosa damascene)..320 MHz
- Joy..189 MHz
- Helicrysum...181 MHz
- Frankincense..147 MHz
- Ravensara...134 MHz
- Lavender (Lavendula angustifolia).......................108 MHz
- Myrrh (Commiphora myrrha)................................105 MHz
- Blue Chamomile (Matricaria recutita)..................105 MHz
- German Camomile...105 MHz
- Blue Tansy...105 MHz
- Melissa...102 MHz
- Juniper (Juniperus osteosperma).............................98 MHz
- Aloes/Sandalwood (Santalum album).....................96 MHz

- Citrus Fresh……………………………………..91 MHz
- Angelica (Angelica archangelica)…………………..85 MHz
- Peppermint (Mentha peperita)……………………..78 MHz
- Galbanum (Ferula gummosa)……………………...56 MHz
- Basil (Ocimum basilicum)………………………...52 MHz
- Purification……………………………………...45 MHz

Most vaccinations are for viruses. The actual vaccine can leave LIVE viruses in your body for YEARS! The following oils will KILL VIRUSES! These may be taken a few drops in a spoonful of honey or a few drops in an empty veggie capsule. They can additionally be dispensed in a room by an essential oil diffuser These also maybe used AFTER the detox to boost the immune system when confronted with a new pathogen.

Any citrus oil

Frankincense

Myrrh

Cinnamon

Lemongrass

Pine Needle

Eucaylptus

Any pine, cypress or spruce

FRUIT

NEARLY ANY FRUIT ACTS AS A DETOX AGENT. FRUITS HAVE MANY ACIDS THAT BREAK DOWN HARMFUL SUBSTANCES. BERRIES HAVE THE NAME "VACCI" IN THEIR LATIN NAME AND ACT AS NATURAL IMMUNE BUILDERS. CITRUS FRUITS INCLUDING BERGAMOT. ALL CONTAIN NATURAL CHEMICALS INCLUDING VITAMIN C THAT DETOX THE BLOOD AND TISSUES. SUPERFRUITS WORK FASTER AT DETOXING THAN OTHER FRUITS.

ACAI

BILBERRIES

BLUEBERRIES

CRANBERRIES

ELDERBERRIES

GOGI BERRIES

MANGO

MANGOSTEEN

PAPAYA

RASPBERRIES

STRAWBERRIES

VITAMINS-

B-100 VITAMINS COMPLEX
VITAMIN C-10,000 MGS ESTER, BUFFERED FORM
VITAMIN D
D-ALPHA VITAMIN E

MINERALS-

SELENIUM- NutriCology Selenium Solution -- 8 fl oz-

ZINC- ADULTS- 21st Century, Zinc Chewable, Cherry Flavored, 90 Chewables

SUPPLEMENTS-

I HAVE CHOSEN CHEWABLES, SQUEEZE PACKETS, AND LIQUIDS THAT ARE THE MOST PLEASANT AND EASIEST TO GET CHILDREN TO TAKE. POWDERS CAN BE STIRRED INTO JUICE, MILK, APPLESAUCE OR YOGURT. ADULTS CAN TAKE THESE ALSO!

DETOX-

-Buried Treasure Bentonite™ Detoxing Formula Peppermint Oil -- 32 fl oz

NERVE BUILDING WHILE DETOXING-

-Buried Treasure Added Attention for Children -- 16 fl oz

-Buried Treasure Neuro-Nectar -- 16 fl oz

PROBIOTICS

PROBIOTICS SHOULD BE CHOSEN NOT BY THE MILLIONS AND BILLIONS NUMBERS BUT BY THE NUMBER OF INDIVIDUAL STRAINS OF PROBIOTICS IN THE SUPPLEMENT. EACH STRAIN DOES SOMETHING DIFFERENT FROM ANOTHER IN THE EFFORT TO PROTECT YOU.

THE BEST COMMERCIALLY AVAILABLE FORMULA IS GARDEN OF LIFE RAW PROBIOTICS FOR WOMEN VAGINAL CARE (MEN AND BOYS CAN TAKE THIS, ALSO!)- ONLY BECAUSE IT IS THE BEST FORMULA ON THE COMMERCIAL MARKET WITH 38 FORMS OF PROBIOTICS! 38! MEN AND CHILDREN CAN TAKE THIS, ALSO. THE CAPSULES CAN BE OPENED AND IT CAN BE STIRRED INTO ANY DRINK INCLUDING A BABY BOTTLE.

Probiotics process and break down harmful substances in your body- so very vital in detoxifying from the injections!

Other choices

- GoLive Kids! Probiotic plus Prebiotic Drink Mix Berry-Licious -- 10 Packet-15 PROBIOTICS

-Garden of Life Dr. Formulated Probiotics Organic Kids Plus Berry Cherry -- 30 Yummy Chewables- 13 PROBIOTICS

-Dr. Mercola Complete Probiotics Powder Packets for Kids Natural Raspberry -- 10 billion CFU - 30 Packets-10 PROBIOTICS

-Renew Life Ultimate Flora™ Kids Probiotic Berry-Licious -- 3 billion - 30 Chewable Tablets!-6 PROBIOTICS

-Garden of Life RAW Probiotics™ Kids -- 3.4 oz!

ENZYMES

- NOW Foods Acid Relief with Enzymes -- 60 Chewables

- Garden of Life Dr. Formulated Enzymes Organic Digest + Tropical Fruit -- 90 Chewables

VITAMIN C-

- Vitacost Vitamin C-500 Natural Fruit Chew Blueberry, Raspberry & Boysenberry -- 500 mg - 180 Chewable Wafers

- Natural Factors 100% Natural Fruit Chew C Blueberry Raspberry and Boysenberry -- 500 mg - 180 Chewable Wafers

- Natural Factors 100% Natural Fruit Chew C Jungle Juice -- 500 mg - 180 Chewable Wafers

COLLOIDAL SILVER-

- VITACOST 500 PARTS PERMILLION COLLOIDAL SILVER

GARLIC-

- FRESH, RAW, ORGANIC

- KYOLIC GARLIC #102

ALL PURPOSE IMMUNE SUPPORT -(to be taken as a detoxifier and in the future when confronted with a pathogen)

- Buried Treasure Prevention ACF -- 16 fl oz LIQUID

- Buried Treasure Children's ACF Immune Support -- 16 fl oz- LIQUID

- Buried Treasure ACF Fast Relief Immune Support -- 16 fl oz- LIQUID

- Source Naturals Wellness Children's Immune Chewable™ -- 60 Soft Chews

- Source Naturals Wellness Immune Chewable™ Berry -- 60 Chewable Wafers

- Enzymatic Therapy Sea Buddies™ -- 60 Chewable Tablets

- DaVinci Laboratories Immuno-DMG™ with Elderberry & Vitamin D3 -- 120 Chewable Tablets

OMEGAS-

- Coromega Orange- LIQUID PACKETS

COLOSTRUM-

Symbiotics Colostrum Plus® Orange

CHLOROPHYLL LIQUID-

Organic Liquid chlorophyll with peppermint or spearmint

DETOX DRINK

- A gallon of distilled water
- 1 cup of organic cranberry juice
- 3 organic fresh lemons
- Liquid stevia and liquid cayenne to taste

ELIMINATE

Alcohol: Alcohol can cause a fatty liver, so it can destroy any detox program you follow.

Caffeinated Beverages: They make the liver work overtime to process the caffeine inside of them, so avoid the beverages with caffeine if you're trying to detox.

Chocolates: Excess sugar means excess stress to your liver. For better cleansing efforts, try to cut out chocolate as well as other sweets and candies

Non organic foods of any kind: the many chemicals on non organic foods only complicate the chemical environment in your body. Organic foods start a natural detox on their own in addition to the supplements you will be taking

ALWAYS DETOX BEFORE BUILDING UP!

ALWAYS DO A PARASITE CLEANSE BEFORE ANY OTHER DETOXING!

DOING A PARASITE CLEANSE-

ALTHOUGH THE VACCINATIONS, IMMUNIZATIONS, AND FLU SHOTS MAY NOT CONTAIN ANY WHOLE OR LIVE PARASITES, THE TOXIC METALS AND CHEMICALS YOU ARE TRYING TO ELIMINATE ARE HELD IN THE BODY IN THE BODY OF THE PARASITES IF THERE ARE ANY PARASITES PRESENT. SO THE FIRST STEP TO GETTING RID OF THE TOXINS IS TO TAKE A PARASITE CLEANSE, THEN THE TOXINS WILL BE ABLE TO BE ELIMINATED MORE READILY. SOME OF THE TOXINS WILL EVEN LEAVE THE BODY IN THE DEAD PARASITE BODIES!

THEN DO A TOXIC METAL CLEANSE.

THEN DO A VIRAL, BACTERIAL, MOLD, AND FUNGAL CLEANSE.

DO LIVER FLUSHES EVERY 3 WEEKS.

DO KIDNEY FLUSHES AT SOME POINT AFTER THE PARASITE CLEANSE.

I urge you to read my foundational book NATURAL HERBAL THERAPY to know all the things you must address to get fully recovered health. Reading this book is like my giving you a 4 hour lecture in the many things that affect our health in this modern world.

THE PLAN

Here is a PLAN for you to follow using all the above information! I will refer to the patient as "him".

All of the supplements mentioned can be taken by adults, also, no matter how long it has been since the last injection.

There will be two parts- the parasite cleanse and then the toxin cleanse. For each part there is a an adult chart to follow for adults and a child chart to follow for children. ALL FOUR CHARTS ARE BASIC OUTLINES FOR A THOROUGH CLEANSE. IF YOU FEEL YOU HAVE A VERY PARTICULAR UNIQUE PROBLEM, YOU MAY CONTACT ME FOR SPECIFIC CHANGES OR ADDITIONS.

The diet should always be organic and mostly vegan for anyone, anytime, and any condition. Your body detoxes on veggie and fruit fiber and chlorophyll and very specific chemicals occurring naturally in herbs. The foods should be mainly the ones on the lists above.

For your child to like being on this plan for several weeks, you should try to make it as comfortable and tasty as possible. Some of the most healing/detoxing herbs are bitter. Adjusting the taste with all organic fruit juices, fruit sauces, honey, maple syrup, stevia, blended dates, coconut sugar, date sugar, etc. can be very helpful. Dark blue grape juice, pomegranate juice, blueberry juice and other dark juices can mask flavors quite well.

STEP ONE

Do a comprehensive parasite cleanse-

PATIENT SCHEDULE

LUCINDA ROBINSON
NATURAL HERBAL THERAPY
815A WYNNSHIRE DRIVE
HICKORY, NC 28601 USA
www.naturalherbaltherapy.info
naturalherbaltherapy@gmail.com
PH# 828-514-2818

SAMPLE CHILD VACCINATION, IMMUNIZATION, FLU NAME
SHOT DETOX
PART 1
ADULT AGES 13 AND ABOVE
PATIENT NAME:

DATE

PRODUCT	WHEN ARISING	BREAKFAST	10:00 AM	LUNCH	3:00 PM	DINNER	BEFORE SLEEP	
PARANIL DR.FLORAS, HUMAWORM OR OTHER		7.		7		7		WWW.DRNATURA.COM OR WWW.VITACOST.COM OR OTHER
ORGANIX NEEM OIL DROPS OR NEEM CAPSULES		2 CAPS OR 2 DROPS				2 CAPS OR 2 DROPS		WWW.VITACOST.COM
500 PARTS PER MILLION COLLOIDAL SILVER		1 t.				1 t.		WWW.VITACOST.COM
BURIED TREASURE ACF		1 T.		1 T.		1 T.		WWW.VITACOST.COM
HIGH CBD CANNABIS OIL		1 t		1 t		1 t		WWW.HEMPWORX.COM
GARDEN OF LIFE RAW PROBIOTICS FOR WOMEN VAGINAL CARE-38 FORMS OR GARDEN OF LIFE DR FORMULATED ORGANIC KIDS CHEWABLE PROBIOTICS		6 /2						WWW.VITACOST.COM 6 THE FIRST DAY AND 2 EVERY DAY THEREAFTER
CASTOR OIL		1 T.						FOR 3 DAYS ONLY

NATURE'S PLUS ORANGE JUICE ESTER, BUFFERED VITAMIN C-CHEWA BLE-1000 MGS.		3,000 MGS		3000 MGS		4,000 MGS		WWW.VITACOST.COM
CHRISTOPHER'S OIL OF GARLIC DROPS OR KYOLIC ODORLESS GARLIC #100 OR #102		2 DROPS OR 2 CAPS				2 DROPS OR 2 CAPS		WWW.VITACOST.COM
GARDEN OF LIFE DR.FORMULATED CHEWABLE DIGESTIVE ENZYMES		1 TO 2				1 TO 2		WWW.VITACOST.COM
		.		.		.		

PATIENT SCHEDULE

LUCINDA ROBINSON
NATURAL HERBAL THERAPY
815A WYNNSHIRE DRIVE
HICKORY, NC 28601 USA
www.naturalherbaltherapy.info
naturalherbaltherapy@gmail.com
PH# 828-514-2818

SAMPLE CHILD VACCINATION, IMMUNIZATION, FLU SHOT DETOX
PART 1
CHILD AGES 1-12
PATIENT NAME:

DATE:

PRODUCT	WHEN ARISING	BREAKFAST	10:00 AM	LUNCH	3:00 PM	DINNER	BEFORE SLEEP	
PARASITE HERBAL FORMULA- DR.CHRISTOPHER LIQUID OR PARANIL ,JR		1 T.				1 T.		WWW.DRNATURA.COM OR WWW.VITACOST.COM
ORGANIX NEEM OIL DROPS		2 DROPS				2 DROPS		WWW.VITACOST.COM
500 PARTS PER MILLION COLLOIDAL SILVER		1/2 t.				½ t.		WWW.VITACOST.COM
BURIED TREASURE ACF		1 T.				1 T.		WWW.VITACOST.COM
HIGH CBD CANNABIS OIL		1 T.				1 T.		WWW.HEMPWORX.COM
GARDEN OF LIFE RAW PROBIOTICS FOR WOMEN VAGINAL CARE-38 FORMS OR GARDEN OF LIFE DR FORMULATED ORGANIC KIDS CHEWABLE PROBIOTICS		6 /2						WWW.VITACOST.COM 6 THE FIRST DAY AND 2 EVERY DAY THEREAFTER
CASTOR OIL		1 t.						FOR 3 DAYS ONLY

NATURE'S PLUS ORANGE JUICE ESTER, BUFFERED VITAMIN C-CHEWA BLE-1000 MGS.	3,000MGS				2,000MGS		WWW.VITACOST.COM
CHRISTOPHER'S OIL OF GARLIC DROPS	2 DROPS				2 DROPS		WWW.VITACOST.COM
GARDEN OF LIFE DR.FORMULATED CHEWABLE DIGESTIVE ENZYMES	1 TO 2				1 TO 2		WWW.VITACOST.COM
	.		.		.		

BECAUSE there are many heavy metals/poisoning chemicals in different vaccinations, and

BECAUSE parasites can cause these heavy metals/poisoning chemicals to be held in the human body inside THEIR bodies,

BECAUSE parasites will continually release these heavy metals/poisoning chemicals in their wastes while alive and dying in your body, and

BECAUSE in the list of things that can tear down your health, parasites are the STRONGEST partners with other things on the list (such as viruses, bacteria, molds, fungi, etc.) THAT CAN ALSO BE IN THESE HARMFUL INJECTIONS, it is IMPERATIVE you do a comprehensive parasite FIRST!

For children- they can take Paranil, Jr. or Dr. Christopher's Parasite Liquid. Older children can take double the dosage. Adults can take Paranil, Parathunder, Humaworm, Scram, Rascal, Herbal Guard, Dr. Floras parasite herbs, etc. I suggest 10 to 21 capsules a day for adults. These kill most native North American parasites. Take 2 neem capsules 2 times a day to kill equatorial and South East Asian parasites, also. This can be taken with any organic baby food, applesauce, fruit juice, or yogurt. They should keep taking it at least 7 days after you see the last parasite or parasite eggs pass in their stool. This may take 6 days or 6 weeks. If you never see anything, do it for at least 3 weeks. If the child can swallow pills or capsules, they should take 2 neem capsules (kills tropical and equatorial parasites) daily, and 1 teaspoon of castor oil for three days ONLY. Adults should take 4 neem capsules a day

THROUGHOUT the detox and 1 tablespoon of castor oil daily for 3 days only.

Because parasites release their stored viruses and bacteria as they die and decompose, you should give your child ½ teaspoon 500 parts per million colloidal silver (tasteless) every time they take the parasite killing herbs. This will kill off the viruses and bacteria as they are released so that your child does not get a short term viral or bacterial infection in the process. If they are older, they can also take 1 teaspoon Buried Treasure ACF with every dose of parasite killing herbs. Also take 1 to 3 teaspoons cannabis oil and colostrum daily if the child has severe autistic spectrum symptoms, seizures, etc. Adults can take the same dosages.

Add 2 capsules daily of Garden of Life Raw Probiotics for Women Vaginal Care- 38 forms of probiotics. Capsules may be opened and mixed with cottage cheese, yogurt, fruit sauce or liquid. Powder from the capsules may be also added to baby bottles. Adults can take 6 capsules the first day to flood the system with probiotics and then 2 capsules every day thereafter.

Children can also take 5000 mgs. ester, buffered Vitamin C daily and adults 10,000 mgs. ester buffered Vitamin C daily in divided doses.

Adults can add 2 caplets, tablets, or capsules of Kyolic garlic 2 or 3 times a day.

If the child is having digestive problems, give him one digestive enzyme product mentioned in the digestive enzyme list for children above with every major meal. Adults can take one or two Garden of Life Raw Enzymes with each meal. Digestive enzymes not only help break down foods, but can also break down some of the unwanted chemicals in the body from the vaccinations as well as undigested colon waste. A DROP OR TWO OF WINTERGREEN OIL IN A SPOONFUL OF HONEY CAN ALSO HELP THE DIGESTION PROCESS OF A SMALL CHILD.

Both adults and children should take 1 to 3 teaspoons of cannabis oil (CBD) daily. This oil deals with pain and nerve transmission problems. It should be the low THC and high CBD type oil that is legal in all 50 USA states.

Frequent B-100 complex tablets and 400 to 600 mgs. of Source Naturals Ultra Mag help re-establish proper nerve transmissions.

This part should last at least 3 weeks. Most parasites, viruses, molds, and bacteria should be eliminated by now.

At day 21, 42, 63, and 84 (or every 3 weeks while on the regimen) take a liver/gallbladder flush.

ONE DAY SIMPLE LIVER FLUSH

THIS MAY BE DONE ONCE BEFORE STARTING A REGIMEN.

DONE 3 WEEKS APART STARTING AT DAY 21 UNTIL DAY 84 (4 DIFFERENT ONE DAY LIVER FLUSHES EACH 3 WEEKS/21DAYS APART) CHILDREN MAY TAKE ½ OR ¼ DOSAGES ACCORDING TO WEIGHT AND AGE CHOOSE A WEEKEND DAY TO DO THIS LIKE A FRIDAY NIGHT OR A SATURDAY NIGHT.

MIX TOGETHER—

3 CUPS WATER OR HOMEMADE FRESH HONEY LEMONADE
4 t. EPSOM SALTS (MAGNESIUM SOURCE)
½ CUP OLIVE OIL
2/3 CUP FRESHLY SQUEEZED PINK GRAPEFRUIT JUICE

MIX ALL TOGETHER AND DIVIDE INTO 4 JARS WITH LIDS. REFRIGERATE.

DO NOT EAT ANYTHING AFTER 4 PM.

AT 4 PM, 6 PM, 8 PM, AND 10 PM DRINK CONTENTS OF ONE JAR.
At 10 PM, ALSO TAKE 10 PARANIL OR DR.FLORAS PARASITE DEFENSE CAPSULES.

GO TO BED WITH HEAD ELEVATED ON ONE OR TWO PILLOWS.

IF YOU WAKE UP IN THE NIGHT, DRINK LOTS OF WATER.

UPON ARISING, DRINK LOTS OF WATER.

YOUR FIRST BOWEL MOVEMENT OF THE DAY SHOULD BE SOFT, GREENISH, AND CONTAIN GALLSTONES AND OTHER LIVER TOXINS AND OTHER

DEBRIS. IF NOTHING HAPPENS, IT WILL ON YOUR SECOND OR THIRD CLEANSE.

REPEAT IN 3 WEEKS AND IN 6 WEEKS AND IN 9 WEEKS AND IN 12 WEEKS UNTIL YOU HAVE DONE A TOTAL OF 4 CLEANSES.

STEP TWO

This next step will eliminate most heavy metals stored in the body.

PATIENT SCHEDULE

SAMPLE ADULT VACCINATION, IMMUNIZATION, FLU SHOT DETOX
PART TWO
ADULT 13 YEARS AND OLDER

PATIENT NAME

DATE

LUCINDA ROBINSON
NATURAL HERBAL THERAPY
815A WYNNSHIRE DRIVE
HICKORY, NC 28601 USA
www.naturalherbaltherapy.info
naturalherbaltherapy@gmail.com
PH# 828-514-2818

PRODUCT	WHEN ARISING	BREAKFAST	10:00 AM	LUNCH	3:00 PM	DINNER	BEFORE SLEEP	
CILANTRO/MORINDA JUICE								ALL DAY
ORGANIC BURDOCK TEA			1 CUP		1 CUP			WWW.VITACOST.COM
NATURE'S WAY CHEWABLE ZINC LOZENGE.		2						
SELENIUM LIQUID-200 MCGS.		X						
CHILDLIFE PROBIOTICS PLUS COLOSTRUM		2						WWW.VITACOST.COM
CARROT JUICE ORGANIC		1 CUP				1 CUP		FRESHLY MADE
HIGH CBD CANNABIS OIL		1 t		1 t		1 t		WWW.HEMPWORX.COM
CHARCOAL CAPS OR POWDER							½ t in liquid	WWW.VITACOST.COM
SIMPLE TRUTH MSM		3000 MGS.						WWW.VITACOST.COM
OREGANO OIL CAPSULES (OPT.)		2						WWW.VITACOST.COM
ORGANIC CHLORELLA POWDER OR TABLETS		2 TO 4						WWW.VITACOST.COM
ORGANIC SPIRULINA POWDER OR TABLETS		2 TO 4						WWW.VITACOST.COM

CHOROPHYLL LIQUID		1 T				1 T		WWW.VITACOST.COM
NATURAL VITALITY ORGANIC LIFE		1 OUNCE						WWW.VITACOST.COM
BLUBONNET EARTH SWEET CHEWABLE-MAGNESIUM		400 MGS						WWW.VITACOST.COM
SOLARAY CHEWABLE B COMPLEX		1		1		1		WWW.VITACOST.COM
CILANTRO JUICE		1 CUP				1 CUP		

Some powders may have to be mixed with liquids, fruit sauces, or yogurt

PATIENT SCHEDULE

SAMPLE CHILD VACCINATION, IMMUNIZATION, FLU SHOT DETOX
PART TWO
CHILD AGES 1-12

PATIENT NAME _____

DATE _____

LUCINDA ROBINSON
NATURAL HERBAL THERAPY
815A WYNNSHIRE DRIVE
HICKORY, NC 28601 USA
www.naturalherbaltherapy.info
naturalherbaltherapy@gmail.com
PH# 828-514-2818

PRODUCT	WHEN ARISING	BREAKFAST	10:00 AM	LUNCH	3:00 PM	DINNER	BEFORE SLEEP	
CILANTRO/MORINDA JUICE								ALL DAY
ORGANIC BURDOCK TEA			1 CUP					WWW.VITACOST.COM
NATURE'S WAY CHEWABLE ZINC LOZENGE.		2						
SELENIUM LIQUID-200 MCGS.		X						
CHILDLIFE PROBIOTICS PLUS COLOSTRUM		2						WWW.VITACOST.COM
CARROT JUICE ORGANIC		1 CUP				1 CUP		FRESHLY MADE
HIGH CBD CANNABIS OIL		1 t		1 t		1 t		WWW.HEMPWORX.COM
CHARCOAL CAPS OR POWDER							½ t in liquid	WWW.VITACOST.COM
SIMPLE TRUTH MSM		3000 MGS.						WWW.VITACOST.COM
OREGANO OIL CAPSULES (OPT.)		2						WWW.VITACOST.COM
ORGANIC CHLORELLA POWDER OR TABLETS		2 TO 4						WWW.VITACOST.COM
ORGANIC SPIRULINA POWDER OR TABLETS		2 TO 4						WWW.VITACOST.COM

CHOROPHYLL LIQUID		1 T				1 T		WWW.VITACOST.COM
NATURAL VITALITY ORGANIC LIFE		1 OUNCE						WWW.VITACOST.COM
BLUBONNET EARTH SWEET CHEWABLE-MAGNESIUM		400 MGS						WWW.VITACOST.COM
SOLARAY CHEWABLE B COMPLEX		1		1		1		WWW.VITACOST.COM
CILANTRO JUICE		1 CUP				1 CUP		
NATURAL VITALITY ORGANIC LIFE		1 OUNCE						WWW.VITACOST.COM

Some powders may have to be mixed with liquids, fruit sauces, or yogurt

Take one whole fresh bunch of organic cilantro, wash, chop, and put in a blender. Add 1 T. organic green morinda powder. Cover with filtered water and blend for at least 1 minute. This should make at least a quart of cilantro/morinda juice mix. You may add any organic juice (carrot, grape, apple, cherry, orange, etc.) if the child objects to the taste. Have the child drink all of this over the whole day. Strain it if it is going into a baby bottle for an infant. He should also take 4 chlorella tablets and 4 spirulina tablets early in the day. These can be chewed or powdered and mixed with juice or any fruit sauce or powdered and added to a spoonful of honey or maple syrup. In the evening, he should drink 1 cup of organic burdock tea. This tea may be sweetened with honey, lemon, maple syrup, or organic stevia and/or organic apple or grape juice added if he objects to the taste.

Older children and adults should take 2 oregano oil capsules a day and 3000 mgs MSM daily to complete the killing of fungi and candida.

50 mgs. zinc gluconate, 200 mgs. selenium, a Coromega Orange packet, 2 T. of chlorophyll liquid, and 500 mgs glutathione daily should be taken by adults.

A few drops of lemon grass oil, pine needle oil or any citrus oil can be put in an empty veggie capsule and taken daily.

COLOSTRUM SHOULD BE TAKEN DAILY UNTIL SYMPTOMS SUBSIDE COMPLETELY

This should be done for 3 weeks.

On day 42, 63, and 84 of this Step Two, give him a one day liver/gallbladder flush to flush the liver, ducts, and gallbladder of all the filtered debris.

Continue the B-100 complex daily and at least 400 mgs. Source Naturals Ultra Mag

You can continue this for another 3 weeks and then do another liver flush.

STEP THREE

By now, you should start seeing some improvements in symptoms. To further improve symptoms, have him take 1 Coromega Orange packet a day and a 30 to 50 mgs. zinc gluconate tablet a day. A charcoal capsule or ½ teaspoon activated charcoal can be taken daily for 3 days in yogurt or fruit sauce. Frankincense oil rubbed anywhere on the body for adults and on the backs and feet of children helps correct many DNA aberrations over time. Drinking noni (morinda fruit) juice and using garlic in cooking and garlic oil in capsules also helps in the process of returning cells to normal functioning. Cannabis oil (CBD) daily by mouth helps with nerve malfunctions and pain. Continue the probiotic capsules indefinitely.

There are some parts of receiving injections with the various poisons and varied undigested DNA that researchers are still not understanding. All we can do is detox those things that can be detoxed. Many have come out with remarkable results when these simple clear steps are taken.

This plan works very well if steps are taken in order. You should see symptoms drop off during each step. The diet plus the supplements should form a healing base and detoxing base for all the received injections.

Dealing with Covid

In dealing with any pathogen, we have Biblical guidelines as to how to cope with them.

We are told to wash our bodies, belongings, and environment frequently in torah (Exodus 12- the end of Deuteronomy).Exodus 30, Leviticus 13-15

We are told to isolate and quarantine anyone with a communicable disease until the disease goes away. For viruses, this is about 3 full weeks, with washing happening during and at the end of the 3 week period. Leviticus 13

We are instructed to wash, throw away, burn, fire clean(sterilize) or bury any infective fabric or surface-like handkerchiefs, tissues, items from other family groups, etc. Numbers 31:23, Leviticus 13-14

In the past, whenever there was a worldwide plague or pandemic, the pathogens always ended up in the ground from washing and toileting, in time. There the soil probiotics broke the pathogen down, rendering it harmless.

In concentrated populations where sewage was not put underground as commanded in torah(Deuteronomy23:13), and animals roamed freely (rats, mice, birds, cats, dogs, hogs, etc.), the animals would pick up the pathogen, store it in their bodies, and then pass it on somewhere to another human. These animals are now called "animal reservoirs". Any scavenger animal or Scripturally defined "unclean"(Leviticus 11 and Deuteronomy 14) or unkosher animal is an animal reservoir as they by nature eat decaying animal and plant materials of any kind. So eating and touching and kissing the unclean animals of the Bible continually sheds and spreads these different toxic pathogens in the population. Deuteronomy 23:13 commands all body waste has to be buried.

Because of the very small size of virus particles, the only masks that can truly protect you are the full hard plastic masks that cover the face (eyes, nose, and mouth) with a charcoal filter. All others are worthless at filtering out viruses!

There are several Scriptural reasons we can not take vaccinations into our bodies.

The first is that aborted fetal cells lines are the backbone of vaccination production. As believers in the Creator, we can not have anything to do with the abortion industry, let alone take these unthinkable cell lines into our bodies.

The second is related to the first in that taking these cell lines into our bodies is akin to cannibalism, an astonishment and abomination in the sight of our Creator.

In addition, we do not know exactly what happens when the female cell line is injected into a male or when a male cell line is injected into a female. This may be one of many reasons we now have gender confusion.

The third is vaccinations contain assorted DNA from many Scripturally unclean animals like horses, monkey, mouse, crab, and more. We are commanded in Leviticus 11 and Deuteronomy 14 to not take these unclean animals into our bodies and at times not even touch them!

The fourth is related to the third reason in that these vaccinations can contain chimera DNA. Chimera DNA is the fused DNA from

2 or more animals.

The fifth reason is we are instructed that are bodies are the temple of the holy spirit. There are many harmful, toxic chemicals and heavy metals in the vaccinations. We can not permit these to be purposely injected into our bodies, harming and LOWERING the effectiveness of our natural immune system, digestive system, nervous system and heart function!

The following are my suggestions to use if you actually test positive for covid-

Organic everything

Vitamin D3-5000 IUS minimum
Zinc gluconate- 50 mgs.
Hydroxychloroquin or natural substitute- PQQ, tonic water, grapefruit
Ivermectin or natural substitute- Pure planet Organic Parasite Cleanse, neem capsules, other herbal parasite formulas
Lemon
Honey
Citrus oils- orange, lemon, tangerine, grapefruit, bergamot
Olbas oil on chest, front and back
Goldenseal tea or capsules
Frankincense oil or capsules
Myrrh oil or capsules
Buried Treasure ACF
Star anise tea or capsules
Eucalyptus oil- a few drops in a spoonful of honey
Sauted garlic cloves
Pine needle oil- 10 drops per capsule
 Lemongrass oil capsules- 5 to 10 drops

Thyme oil in capsules- 2 to 5 drops
Oregano oil capsules
Any cypress or spruce oil in capsules- 5 to 10 drops
Any Source Naturals Wellness formula
Elderberry syrup
10 grams or 10,000 mgs ester or buffered Vitamin C daily
Cinnamon and ginger tea
Grape juice

Although I am totally opposed to getting any vaccinations whatsoever, here is a list of natural things Dr. Judy Mikovitz, the world's leading authority on viruses and vaccines, says can detox MOST of the ingredients in the covid vaccinations.

No GMO anything, but do eat organic only

Zinc-50 mgs.
Vitamin D- 5000 IUS minimum
Hydroxychloroquin or natural substitutes- PQQ, tonic water, grapefruit
Ivermectin or natural substitues- neem, Pure Planet Organic Parasite Cleanse and others
Quercetin
NAC or n-acetyl-cysteine
DMG or di-methyl glycine-breaks up MRNA
SAM-adenosyl-L-methione
Glutathione, glycine or Pro-Immune
Magnesium or Magnesium Breakthrough
Selenium
Low dose interferon spray
Chicken soup
Cannabinoids-CBD-skin balm
Ozonated skin creams

Get good sleep-melatonin, lavender oil on feet
Turn off all 5G wifi at night
Stop fear and anger as it stops immune system
Light therapy- 30 minutes in the sun daily
No masks

I would add 10 grams ester or buffered Vitamin C, garlic, frankincense, myrrh, pine needle oil, pomegranate, hemp, noni or morinda for DNA repair

VACCINE, IMMUNIZATION, FLU SHOT EDUCATION WEBSITES-

- Vaccine Truth
- VACINFO.ORG
- Think Twice
- Vac Truth
- Vac Facts
- Vax Truth
- Vaccination Liberation
- The Story Behind The Story
- Educate-Yourself
- WHALE
- Vaccination News
- VaccineInjury.info
- Childhoodshots.com
- KOREN Publications
- Crusador
- WAVE (World Association for Vaccine Education)
- PROVE (Parents Requesting Open Vaccine Education)
- The Doctor Within
- PAVE (People Advocating Vaccine Education)
- HAPI (Health Advocacy in the Public Interest)
- Medicina Alternativa
- Vacunacion Libre
- ZEUS
- Vaccine Associated Sarcoma
- Canine Health Concerns
- Peaceful Pregnancy Pathways

ESSENTIAL OILS THAT KILL PATHOGENS-

THIS LIST MAY BE USED AFTER THE DETOX TO CONTINUALLY HELP THE IMMUNE SYSTEM DEAL WITH NEW INCOMING PATHOGENS

BERGAMOT

CINNAMON

CLOVES

EUCALYPTUS

GRAPEFRUIT

LEMON

LEMONGRASS

MYRRH

ORANGE

OREGANO

PINE OIL

TANGERINE

SPRUCES

ABOUT THE AUTHOR AND CONTACT INFORMATION

Lucinda Robinson is an herbalist since 1973 from Hickory, North Carolina, USA. She is a Messianic/Nazarene Israelite believer. She was called by YAHUAH in 1967 and gave her life to Him in faith and obedience in June of 1970. She is married to David and has 8 grown children and 10 grandchildren. She attended Cornell University where she studied child development, nutrition, consumer advocacy, and communications. She home birthed 7 of her children and homeschooled all 8 children for a total 14 years. She loves to study nutrition, herbal and natural cures for disease, the use of essential oils for healing, the history of the paganization and heathenization of the church, the true role of women from a Scriptural perspective, home industries, Scriptural archeology, the 4,000 plus year history of Messianic Judaism, the history of dress and dress design, organic gardening, and vegan cooking and raw food preparation.

Lucinda helps individuals in their homes or care facility to address their chronic and critical health needs as a natural health care worker as well as gives lectures and seminars on health and women's spiritual issues. She is a women's torah teacher.

Other books by Lucinda are available on www.amazon.com as well as the website-www.naturalherbaltherapy.info.

She counsels by appointment at her office and by phone (828-514-2818), e-mail, and regular mail. You may contact her by e-mail at naturalherbaltherapy@gmail.com, by phone and Skype at natural.herbal.therapy, or by mail at 815 A Wynnshire Drive, Hickory, North Carolina, 28601 USA. Her foundational book, NATURAL HERBAL THERAPY, and more information is available at her website- www.naturalherbaltherapy.info.

Lucinda Robinson is not medical doctor and has never claimed to be a medical doctor. Every client asking for help comes with a medical doctor's diagnosis in hand before counseling can start. Lucinda does not diagnose. She is an herbalist counseling clients about the well known, publicly published, and proven natural treatments that have proven over many years to be effective for certain health problems using herbs, vitamins, minerals, enzymes, probiotics, and other non-invasive physical treatments. Lucinda takes no responsibility for any effects that may come from anyone trying her suggested treatments and their results in that particular person. There are so many variable possibilities that affect health that an absolute certain outcome can not be guaranteed, especially if they are not under Natural Herbal Therapy's counseling's direct contact and supervision.

Made in the USA
Monee, IL
16 September 2022